MW01231074

FINDING YOUR LIGHT

The Six Healing Paths

SHELLY R. FOX

BALBOA.PRESS
A DIVISION OF HAY HOUSE

Copyright © 2024 Shelly R. Fox.

All rights reserved. No part of this book may be used or reproduced by any means, graphic, electronic, or mechanical, including photocopying, recording, taping or by any information storage retrieval system without the written permission of the author except in the case of brief quotations embodied in critical articles and reviews.

Balboa Press books may be ordered through booksellers or by contacting:

Balboa Press
A Division of Hay House
1663 Liberty Drive
Bloomington, IN 47403
www.balboapress.com
844-682-1282

Because of the dynamic nature of the Internet, any web addresses or links contained in this book may have changed since publication and may no longer be valid. The views expressed in this work are solely those of the author and do not necessarily reflect the views of the publisher, and the publisher hereby disclaims any responsibility for them.

The author of this book does not dispense medical advice or prescribe the use of any technique as a form of treatment for physical, emotional, or medical problems without the advice of a physician, either directly or indirectly. The intent of the author is only to offer information of a general nature to help you in your quest for emotional and spiritual well-being. In the event you use any of the information in this book for yourself, which is your constitutional right, the author and the publisher assume no responsibility for your actions.

Any people depicted in stock imagery provided by Getty Images are models, and such images are being used for illustrative purposes only. Certain stock imagery © Getty Images.

Print information available on the last page.

ISBN: 979-8-7652-5253-6 (sc)
ISBN: 979-8-7652-5254-3 (hc)
ISBN: 979-8-7652-5252-9 (e)

Library of Congress Control Number: 2024910130

Balboa Press rev. date: 06/28/2024

I am so grateful to my family, friends, and spirit team, especially to Amaranth and Amia, who guided me during this process.

To those who have helped me find my own light or helped direct my path, thank you. You have no idea how you have changed my life.

To Candice and Tiff, owners of Indiglow Soul and Essentially Tiff, having you on this healing journey as friends, supporters, and healers has been amazing!

With so much love,
Shelly

Contents

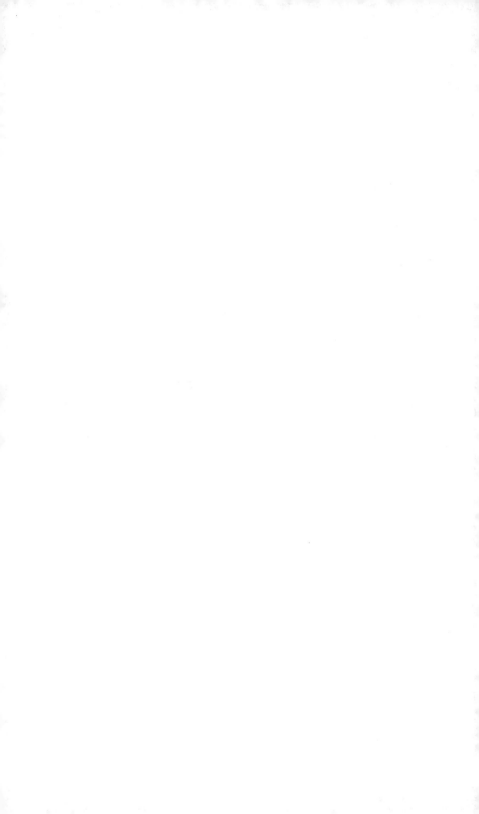

Preface

As little as five years ago, I was oblivious to spiritual awakenings, self-work, twin flames, Reiki, meditation, or that I had a spirit family of amazing beings. I was miserable trying to figure out the right time to give up on my current life. I had a beautiful home, a husband, three dogs, and a secure job. I was trying to focus on holding everything together, but there was a part of me that had given up a year earlier.

A year before this moment, I had made myself a promise that I did not keep. I had let myself down and experienced another round of the same events I swore I would not subject myself to again.

I was so disconnected and sad that I used to cry and pray myself to sleep. I had no idea what to do. I had asked for us to go to therapy, suggested he talk to his friends, family, a pastor, but the drinking just continued until nine days before I was prepared to leave in 2017.

There I was counting down the days until I would get out of the loop when he walked in and announced all I had ever hoped for: his drinking days were over.

Nine months later, I was in an even worse place. I hated how much work our yard and house required; I felt exhausted. I'd been married for fifteen years, and I don't think we even knew each other or ourselves. So here I was, celebrating yet another birthday. (I *hated* my birthday; he always found a way to ruin it for me.) We were sitting in the parking lot at Academy Sports when I stopped holding everything together.

I finally said out loud that I wanted to leave a year earlier and that I had checked out a long time before that. It was a small thing that day, we were simply headed to buy me a pair of sneakers for my birthday, and he started the same thing he did every birthday. I don't have a lot to spend, he would always say, and, seriously, I've been in this relationship for eighteen years, my entire adult life. We both had great jobs and an amazing house, and he couldn't buy a birthday present. A pair of sneakers was too much after I'd dealt with his drunk ass for eighteen years.

I tapped out. I had nothing left to give, and I had no idea what to do. I made a therapy appointment.

Four visits later, I moved out.

And so began my healing journey, which included twin-flame healing. If any of you know much about this type of journey, you know it's no cakewalk. This is how I've spent the last five years. Meeting or connecting with your twin flame kicks off healing for you both and can trigger a spiritual awakening.

So how did this five-year journey go? Well, first, it's still going. Healing is never really complete. I experienced all kinds of adventures and emotions—healing, love, anger, sadness, hope, struggles, beautiful moments, bliss, wonder, awe, frustration, pain, loss, and heartbreak. I also got to know myself. The real me. The one without all the programming, the karma, and the past life trauma. What do I need? What do I want? How do I let go of what no longer serves me? I've read books, watched programs, and continued therapy (therapist number four is a keeper). I had all kinds of sessions—palm readings, card readings, yoga, meditation, Reiki, Emotion/Body Code, shamanic healings and journeys, and even lymphatic drainage. I've been able to meet my spirit guides and so much more.

Can I tell you how much of what we don't understand is karma, past lives, and trauma we don't even remember? Can I tell you how much I've changed, including my belief system? Can I tell you how much hearing, listening to, and loving yourself is so critical to your mind, body, and spiritual health?

Healing is a lot of work, but so worth it because you are meant to feel joy, love, peace, relaxation, and sheer bliss. Magic is real, and so are fairies and dragons and treasure hunts.

Today, I still have the same job I did in 2017, but everything else in my life is more alive, magical, and healthier than it ever was.

Chapter 1

WHY HEALING IS IMPORTANT

We are beings of light who are meant to experience such joy, wonder, and awe. Our past experiences weigh us down, affect our perspectives, change how we react, and unless we heal from these experiences, they continue to shape our reactions. We build walls, hide from shame, avoid conversations, avoid being uncomfortable, or even strive to make others happy. We, in turn, lose ourselves, no longer able to trust our own thoughts and struggle to even decide what it is we want.

We are constantly taught that others can make better choices for us—parents, teachers, religion, friends, family, TV, and even strangers. We search the internet for answers when the answer is within ourselves. You are the best and most qualified person to make decisions for yourself, but if unhealed, the decisions that you make are so skewed from who you really are that it becomes very confusing. In being lost we search for help. Help is tricky because others also have trauma and experiences and even rules, jealousy, and manipulation that play into the help they offer.

So you can see why healing is important, but where in the world do you start when karma, contracts, past lives, and every moment until now has played a part in where you are today?

Let's be clear that the journey you seek is not an easy one: there are no maps, no short cuts, and no secret doors that lead to the end of the work, but knowing yourself, trusting yourself, and loving yourself completely changes your perspective. Imagine making all your decisions from a healed place—influenced by only you and feeling like you have the entire universe and a team of beings all working for your highest and best.

Focus for just a minute; can you picture yourself taking just one step toward healing? That's all it takes: one single step at a time, becoming more and more sure of yourself, uncovering who you are, what you believe, your path, your purpose. Stepping into your power, taking control of your life, no longer making decisions based on what anyone else wants or needs, focused on you. Amazing, gifted, beautiful, present *you*. Are you willing to work hard to find yourself? Are you ready to let go of programming, training, people pleasing, overthinking, anxiety, stress, frustration, and making the best of your current situation? Then do it: take one step, try one thing, look back on one thing, and ask yourself, Can I trust myself?

I couldn't. I'd let myself down so many times, made so many promises that I'd broken. I thought so many other people were better at making decisions, and here I was: a failure at marriage, living in an apartment alone, completely lost with no space to be outside in nature, no comfort from my pets, and an elusive twin flame—classic runner/chaser.

Yoga. A lady from work invited me to a yoga class that was five minutes away from my apartment. It was one day a week, and I could say I socialized and exercised. I was clearly stressed, since my hair was falling out, I'd lost way too much weight, and there was this persistent rash around my nose. My body had held off for so long, and it no longer could. Even tears, I could no longer hold those back. Yoga was a gateway; I received my first crystal and my first exposure to chakras. I can't say that I was really vibing with the whole chakra thing. I clearly remember laying on my back breathing in and out and the teacher asking, What does your third eye need? And mine, it wanted donuts. Fortunately, I've since figured out my third eye is not my stomach, but these classes got me redirected to healing.

Healing, the path is not linear. It looks more like a child's coloring book. All out of the lines, one might even call it ugly. It's vulnerable, sad, exciting, and exhilarating, but hang on: the ride is worth it. Yoga led to a tarot-card and palm reading, which led to Meeting Your Spirit Guide classes, which led to Reiki, which led to Emotion

Code and pendulum work, which led to meditation and journaling, and like following breadcrumbs, I found my way back to myself—the stripped-away version with new beliefs, new wants, new plans, a purpose, and passion.

I can recall sitting in my new apartment living room and a friend asking, "What are you passionate about?" I just remember thinking, *Dude, I don't even know who I am anymore, since I don't live at this address with the beautiful yard, and I'm no longer a wife, and I no longer have the house, the yard, and all the things I've spent the last twenty years chasing. What am I passionate about? I can barely keep myself together, and I have no clue what the fuck I'm passionate about. I've been riding numb for about ten years now.*

Now, five years later, I tell you with all kinds of excitement that I am so passionate about helping others find their light after finding my own and working to keep it lit. I wish I could tell you that it has all been rainbows and unicorns, but there have been many "cocoon" periods, and I'm not always sure that a butterfly is what emerged, but it's *me*—I'm passionate, I believe in magic and miracles and a higher power, and I feel like I'm supported by an amazing team of beings who help me feel like a badass most days. I've found my purpose, my calling, and I can't wait until it's what I get to do every day—to be able to see people find themselves, to uncover who they are and who they want to be. Pastors told my parents that I'd be a healer, that one of their children would break generational curses, but I had no idea that it could be me. So healing is super hard work—physically, mentally, spiritually, and emotionally—but, y'all, I've got to say that it's totally worth it.

So how do you approach healing? Well, there is no one-stop shop, but I do believe there are some crucial steps or elements to healing, six paths to walk on for healing.

intuition
love
nature
conscious/collective
purpose
health

And there are a few cheats, yes; I recall saying that there are no secret passages, but there are a few places in which clues are available. These include your mission animal, your life path number/soul number, and your gifts. We will dive deeper into these concepts, but all six paths are critical to your healing and understanding your gifts and purpose.

For these you can also find a number of online resources.

To find your life path number/master number, add your eight digit birthday together, and keep adding until you have a single number.

To find your mission animal, meditate and ask your mission animal to come forward. What is this animal, and what does it represent?

Your path, purpose, and gifts will emerge if you continue to work on your healing.

Everyone believes in something different, so apply what you believe. I believe there is a higher power, and I view it as the Creator. From this Creator are the six types of healing, and each person must work through and use all six. One of them will resonate more than the others, and this is where you will find your gift. Your gift is your medicine. You'll use your medicine to heal yourself and may also help others too. Your mission animal helps with the implementation of your gift. Your life path number provides the main lesson you have for this lifetime.

Chapter 2

THE PURPOSE OF UNDERSTANDING YOUR PATH

What you came in this world to do will feel like nothing else. It's like the right combination of numbers being entered into a lock and having access to the treasure. It's like working with the ocean, swimming with the currents, using the power of a mighty force: you just enjoy the ride.

A path is typically depicted as one to the left and one to the right, a crossroads. But what if the path is a forest of trees, and you get to make the path? Along the way you may stay a little longer in some spots, so you make it comfortable—perhaps you even return to a beautiful spot because it calls to you, and maybe you end up in an area with quicksand. Well, healing is like that. Some moments feel like the most beautiful, amazing accomplishments, but sometimes something turns your world upside down, and you go back into a cave for safety, rest, and protection.

A path through a forest does not have luxury hotels, hot water, or five-star meals; it has natural beauty where you learn to appreciate the simplest of experiences. Trust that you are on the right path and know that it leads to your purpose and your passion. Continue to find things and people that light your fire, keep moving, stay curious, and it will propel you forward.

Your life is meant to be magical and wonderful, simple and honest, interesting and boring, and prepare you for your purpose. There are parts that will test you, cause you pain, make you reconsider, but what if during your travel while living this life you are simply training for your purpose. If you understand the value of hardship, the lesson, does it make it easier?

I think so. When I realize that someone in my life is simply playing the role within our karmic contract, I learn to appreciate the role they are playing and how good of a job they are doing.

Does everyone have a path? Yes.

Can you choose to pursue it or not? Yes.

Does pursuing it mean you have to heal? Absolutely!

But what if you are all good, no healing required? I have yet to meet anyone like that, so please reach out to me to explain how you tackled every inner child, mother/father experience, trauma, and programming that you've encountered, as, for most, healing is a constant daily practice of working on oneself.

So what are the steps to finding your path/purpose? There isn't one way, but some key places to start with a therapist or healers include the following:

> past lives
> current life regression
> karma and karmic contracts
> inner child
> relationship style and issues
> programming and beliefs that are no longer true
>> for you
> mother/father work
> trauma

What things in life do you struggle with?

Where are you not asking for what you want and need?

Make a list of all your triggers or the things that irritate you about others.

Where are you hard on yourself?

What causes stress or irritation in your life?

How is work? What about your relationships, friends, and health?

Do you work, play, and rest?

What do you dream about doing?

This is not a simple or fast process. Your body can only process so many things at once. Be aware that once you make a consistent effort to heal, your body, mind and spirit will all begin to align and work toward that goal of healing. Some things will even seem like they are getting worse; they are—they are saying, Hey there, it's time to work on me.

Why is your path/purpose connected to your healing? We were designed to be healthy, happy, beautifully aligned beings using our highest and best self to make decisions. But we are all people, and well, people aren't perfect. We make mistakes, and we think with our egos, our trauma, what we've seen others do, and what we saw our parents do.

What we see, hear, and experience all come together to tell us what to do, what to value, and what to strive for. We are taught to ignore our own intuition and accept that someone outside of us knows better than we do. Because Jill looks like she has it all together, she must have it all figured out. Because doing X gets us more praise, more attention, feeds our craving for what is missing from ourselves, that must be what we focus on.

If there is one thing I've learned on my journey—well, two things really—it's that no one knows what I need better than a healed me, and getting directions from TV, social media, friends, family, and so on is very tricky because they also are coming at it from an unhealed place. Even with the best therapist and healers, they are only bumpers on the path to knocking down the pins. You've got to throw the ball down the lane and give it enough force to make it to the end.

Evolution of the soul, which is the purpose of many lifetimes. One soul—different birth times, places, situations, relationships, and lessons. To learn from your past lives, you can use mediation, past life regression sessions, hypnosis, and Akashic records readings. Astrology provides information about your birth time and the personality that you came into this lifetime with. Karmic contracts determine which lessons are not ones you can get out of. In most readings, when I've inquired about my path, I was commonly told, "The road is long and bumpy," and well, I suppose all roads are. My road has been bumpy. I tend to think of the story of *The Princess and the Pea*, where no matter how many mattresses and cushions were used, she could feel the pea.

Well, it seems that ten amazing things can't overshadow one sucky thing with me. Here is where I tell you about the thing I still struggle with: trust.

This journey of healing requires trust in yourself and intuition. Which sounds super easy because I know myself and if I can trust anyone, it's me. It turns out that I had not been able to trust myself for a long time, so even trusting me was complicated. To lean into what you hear when it defies your logic or ego is truly a task difficult to master. I believe that trusting myself is connected to loving myself, and to be honest, knowing me proved to be more challenging than I ever expected.

I was raised in a typical middle-class family. I think most of us think our family is typical. Is anything typical?

We see other families, and we have an idea of what we think they have or do or how easy or hard it looks, but truthfully, you only know the one you have, and you don't really know them. I've been living with myself, well, since I was a baby, and it turns out that I'm not sure I always know me. I was raised Christian via my parents, going to church and a Christian school until eighth grade. It was black and white on many subjects, and frankly, I never put much thought into questioning the religion, politics, or rules of my family unit. For the rules I could not stick to I simply hid those things, which for those of you who have read any Brene Brown, welcome to *shame*. I spent most of my time thinking I was doing a pretty good job of tackling life, a house, a great job, a car, and making enough money to make life easy, but something was not working.

Two people living together with no healing happening were not likely to yield to until death do us part. I think the book *Scary Close* by Donald Miller was the first crack in the wall, the one I'd been holding my fingers in to try to keep things together. It talked about being vulnerable, and there was something about that word. That word would be my life raft for the next two years.

After moving out, I decided that I wanted whatever "vulnerable" was. (Truth be told, I was raw.) I was sitting in the apartment, and there were some rough moments, but I'd always come back to wanting to learn to be vulnerable. I needed to learn to share my feelings and talk to someone. See, I went for over eight years in a tough situation with my husband and I never had one conversation with anyone about how I felt or what I was dealing with. I never went to an in-law, a friend, or a family member or asked for help. I just kept praying since he would not go to therapy. I had prayed for so long that I was pretty sure no one was listening. But looking back, I think the person who needed to respond was me.

This girl is a reformed perfectionist, and the last thing I wanted with my perfect house, perfect yard, and perfect life was a black mark. Divorce literally took every single bit of pride away from me, and I did not know who and what I identified as anymore. Well, folks, I can tell you that losing my pride helped me find vulnerability. Did you know that sharing who you really are and what is really going on with you attracts others? It turns out that people seem to like people who are honest. Crazy, right?

Showing people who you truly are is vulnerable, courageous, and challenging. People need to feel safe before sharing too much and it needs to be within a supportive, healthy friendship. Here is where I tell you that having a good, trustworthy, loving circle of friends is very important. These people need to be healthy, trusting, vulnerable individuals who understand that your decisions are not logical and that they don't need to follow anyone's expectations.

Note that expectations are tricky.

We are taught that high standards are important but high expectations lead us to disappointment. While I know not everyone needs a community, I do truly believe every person needs a few people who they can talk to, share what is going on, and when shit hits the fan, who can help in some way until your response is more relaxed and you can think for yourself. Healing work brings up many things you did not even know you believed.

One day, I was just sitting at my desk working. Out of nowhere I hear, "You don't even believe that you deserve a loving relationship." Well, you have my attention now. Understand that at this point I had been in therapy for five years, and out of my marriage for the same amount of time, doing self-work constantly, and I believe what? So frustrating. It initially felt like a setback. But after moving past the frustration of it, I could easily say, "This needs to go," and ask my team how we get rid of this thought process or belief because it no longer serves my highest and best. Now, logic would dictate that since I started therapy during my separation and divorce, this little tidbit of information would have surfaced and been taken care of early on. But, hey, that's healing; it's not linear, logical, or ever fully done because we continuously heal over the course of our lives. Now that I am aware of this belief and thought process, I can do something about it. Woo-hoo!

What does healing have to do with your purpose? Everything. Your purpose is tied to what drives you. Your purpose is your passion. Your passion lights your path. Your path is only for you, no one can show you a map, but like a treasure hunt, you can be helped along the way.

As a kid, did you ever blindfold yourself and try to find things? It's not very easy; with the blindfold, it's clumsy. Healing is like that; trauma and your experiences are like wearing a blindfold. Choosing to heal is like taking it off and seeing for the first time.

One of my most memorable moments that pointed me to my path was while I was driving. I had finally made the decision to divorce my husband after eight difficult years. I was driving home from work, and it was like I'd been wearing a visor that prevented me from seeing anything above my eye level until that day. I recall thinking, *When did tree trunks get leaves?* It's crazy, but while in an unhealthy situation, I was barely experiencing what was around me because my focus had become so narrow. I've heard of others having a similar experience.

Just one choice, one change, one thought, can start you on the path to doing something for you, and your body, your mind, and your spirit will take notice.

Light. Ever notice how even a little bit of light can change everything? Low light during a dinner romantic. A bright sun, and you cover your eyes. On a hunt in a closet, and you'd love to have a spotlight. Light is great, but the right light is unbelievable.

I was outside one sunny day standing at the door of my garage confused. I knew my husband was hiding something, but I just could not figure it out. I'd checked his bathroom cabinet, his office, and his area in the garage, but my brain knew the math was not adding up. As I stood in the doorway, I saw what almost looked like a spotlight coming down from the sky that pointed its beam on the driver's side door of his work car, so I opened it. This was the first time I knew someone, or something, was helping me. It's hard to believe it now, but that did not even phase me. Discovering what my spouse was hiding from me was my new focus. The next time I had a sign I was peeing at a friend's house, so understand that these things can occur anywhere, anytime, and about anything.

Your body is built to protect itself. During trauma, the human brain can even forget that something occurred while the heart and the body remember. It will still have a tremendous impact on your body, even if you cannot recall the details. Your body stores memories and emotions that could not be released because your body was unable to process them. These emotions can cause health issues. Health issues and physical pain can be a result of physical, emotional, spiritual, or mental causes. Healing requires evaluating all these as well. The "physical symptoms" can be physical, emotional, spiritual, or mental. They can also be a combination of these. Picture a ball of yarn—that gives you a better picture of healing and how complicated it can be. There are many ways to go about healing, but there are six key elements I've used: intuition, love, nature, purpose, conscious/collective, and health. These are the six healing paths. All must be walked, but one of these is where your purpose lies.

Chapter 3

FINDING YOUR PATH/PURPOSE

Your path is not one way, meaning there are many ways to the same place. Your life and the detours it will take decide the route. Healing takes recovery time. Recovery can look different for everyone. It can be sleeping, resting, getting outside, discussions, and sometimes distractions taking off the focus for a short time. Your body and mind also must adjust to the changes. Emotions and trauma that are not released can exist in the body; they can be anywhere. Your systems have been working around the blocks, dams, or general sludge since they occurred. If you experience learning about them via meditation, hypnosis, or dreams, you may see them as items you recognize but not typically found in the human body.

During my healing experience, I've seen my blocks as a piece of wood with nails covering my heart, a wooden peg leg, a refrigerator in my intestines—all of these are not the actual items there but representations of the issue and the block. Fortunately, there are many ways to remove and release these emotions and blocks. What works for you may not work for someone else. The same way in which a song can bring one person to tears while another one hearing it has no clue what it is about, healing and the techniques used are very personal.

I learned an interesting lesson during my process. I always viewed palm readings and tarot-card readings as entertainment; now I understand the value of the information or puzzle pieces they can provide and recognize them as another way to provide hints for direction in healing.

So what does finding your path and purpose bring? It's a feeling of being supported, at peace, and an understanding that finding yourself is the most important task in your life. Making decisions from a healed place allows grace for you and others. I find it so much easier now to remember that what others tend to direct at me has little to do with me and is more about how they feel about themselves. Knowing myself allows me to trust myself and provides the confidence to make decisions and trust that the universe is supporting my growth and healing.

Imagine if you interacted with everyone using your highest and best self with no ego or revenge but just from a healed place, calm, at peace, and difficult to ruffle. Much like a dog turns its head from side to side when a person talks, as if trying to understand, so will you begin to do when another human acts out. Instead of stoking the fire, your ego smothers. You take a deep breath, and you go about your day understanding that they have more healing to do and likely so do you. Meditation, intuition, healing, and knowing your path/purpose all lower anxiety, reduce overthinking, allow you to process the world around you, and help you read your body and what it needs, then provide it to yourself.

Your main path/purpose is one of the six we discussed previously, but healing is brought about when using all six. It will take a while to figure out which of the paths is your main path. However, once your main path appears, keep in mind that any time you are working to heal, considering them all is important, then your gifts will begin to emerge.

For example, if your main path is intuition, then you may work to become an energy healer who uses one or more of the "clairs" to provide guidance and insight during a Reiki session.

In some cases, you will also find that you lost this path early on. In my case, I could hear the thoughts of others as a child, and therefore, my body's protection mechanism included blocking my spiritual ears. I'm clairaudient.

It has taken years of practicing intuition and many sessions of hypnosis to remove this protection mechanism so that I could use my full gift of clairaudience. My main way of working during healing sessions today is hearing. Because I am an empath, and because the thoughts of others prevented me from feeling safe in a home environment, my body enabled systems to protect me. My life experiences and path have led me to working through the trauma via inner-child work, therapy about my father, and using my gifts of intuition. My divorce drove me to search for something other than the typical American dream, and my fascination with palm readers and tarot-card readers, even as a kid, led me to my path/ purpose, all via healing.

What makes someone want to heal? I think it can be any number of things. Physical pain is a big one; however, having the energy to tackle healing is difficult during those periods. The loss of someone you love is another life event that forces one to reconsider what is important and what is not.

Is it frustration, disappointment, confusion, loss of identity, or divorce, or just simply having the knowledge that something needs to change?

Change. Most of us would say that we don't like change. Yet change is what brings about growth, healing, searching, and being willing to go where you have not been willing to go before. Interesting. They say that insanity is doing the same thing over and over and expecting a different response. So changing one thing and watching as a different outcome occurs is that what causes people to continue to be willing to grow and heal. Both growth and healing require some level of getting uncomfortable so one can see and evaluate what doing something different really changes.

I suppose that getting uncomfortable is needed and that something new does feel different. Being open to difference and change does make it easier. When I got divorced, everything changed except for my job. My address changed; I started living alone, going from a house with a yard to an apartment. No longer a wife, no longer a homeowner, and no longer with another person to share the details of my day. Everything except for my clothes and job was different. To say it was uncomfortable was an understatement. I knew things needed to change, but was this what I meant by it? A lot of time alone with new hobbies to keep me busy and no more yard work allowed for a lot of thinking and reading. I stayed in therapy after I left my husband, and I read a lot of self-help books.

If this was my chance to start over, what did I want? Pets? More religion? A boyfriend? I also realized that my life was so tied up in my dogs, my husband, our home and my job that I was left without a whole lot to do. I exercised. I drank. See, I had not had the opportunity to drink in a long time. I even skipped cooking often, which before happened daily. So between being alone, cereal for dinner, and the occasional bottle-of-wine dinner I managed to drop a few pounds, a lot of hair, and picked up a stress nose rash. Life was feeling pretty good—not really.

Fast forward through the next fifteen months and while some things were awesome, some things just sucked. I missed having a house with a yard and some space. I'd started metaphysical classes and then just months later, the school closed. This was my bright spot, and now what? Then COVID-19 hit. I bought a house, got it all set up, and my boyfriend dumped me. The AC went out seven times, the thermostat quit, my job messed up both my federal and state taxes, and to be honest, if one more thing happened, I was pretty sure I was going to throw in the towel.

Fortunately, the lady who taught metaphysical classes at the school started teaching online classes. This changed my life. Then after a one-day class I was going to take was canceled due to COVID-19, one of the teachers offered one free session. A life coach. Sure, I wasn't kicking ass and taking names, so perhaps a life coach could point me in the right direction. I'd tried three therapists and was not getting to the root of my issues. Trying anything new was my motto.

So the life coach's advice was to become very comfortable alone. So much so that you are stingy giving another your time. I had already been doing a lot on my own, and I must tell you, I rolled my eyes more than once during the session.

But she was so right!

I spent the next two years focused on myself and my healing with an amazing new therapist. I kept taking classes and started getting trained in various healing modalities and really put in time doing the work to get to know myself. Now let me say, I have not liked all that I have learned about myself, but my life is so magical, and my direction and outlook have changed so much that I don't even recognize that person from five years ago.

I'm a badass healer who is fully committed to healing myself and others. I have a supportive, amazing group of friends who are unbelievable. I have a life I love. And me by myself—well, if it's that way it ends up until the end of time, I'm OK with that too. I listen to my intuition, to my body, and to my spirit team, and the universe shows me daily that it has my back. I feel fully supported in my healing, my path, and my purpose. I love the people I get to work on and with. Every day I feel so blessed. My attitude of "this is happening to me" has changed to "this is happening *for* me," at least most days.

How have I used the six paths?

Intuition

I started with a simple palm reading and tarot-card reading just hoping for some direction, as many of the things I'd tried or built kept falling apart. This reading mentioned the voice/light from the doorway of the garage and the restroom I mentioned earlier. The spirit world does not recognize personal space. I took classes to get to know this voice and over the course of four years, learned to mediate, met my spirit team, which contains over thirty amazing beings, became certified in four healing modalities, got to be a part of some fantastic local communities, and am now writing this book. I use my intuition daily and work as a healer nearly every day in some way. And just five years ago, I had never been exposed to any of this. Today, I use intuition to figure out what my body needs and what direction I should go in.

Love

Man, oh man! So much love for myself and so much compassion and empathy for others. I spent so much time being angry at my husband and blaming him for what happened, and now I just wish I would have been able to apply what I now know. Through therapy, meditation, journaling, hypnosis, and many other healing modalities, I learned to listen to myself, that I am the expert on what I should do and what I need. My body requires me to take care of me. I remember the moment that I moved from expecting others to heal me, love me, and be a refuge for me to the epiphany that I needed to listen to me, I needed to love me, and I needed to be a refuge for me. If I'm not listening to me, why would anybody else? Self-love is so important to healing.

Conscious/Collective

Caring about other people. I'd say that five years ago, this was not one of my virtues. It is important for me to understand that people come from an unhealed place and remember that most of what others do to me is more about them. Well, craisin! I say craisin when something blows my mind. This year, I volunteered within a community to help with a festival to expose others to this world of healing. I'm a part of a local organization that holds mindful retreats and ceremonies, I own a business that provides healing sessions and classes, and I'm a part of many of the communities within my area just to be with awesome, mindful, talented, healing people. And me, I want to help others; well, if that doesn't say what healing can do, I don't know what does.

Nature

So even before I knew what meditation was, a reader told me I was already doing it. She said you use the outdoors to meditate. When you spend time outside, you work through things going on in your life and determine how you should proceed. Yes, I do move outside when I need to think. I love yard work, sunbathing, and seeing and hearing the ocean. The outside has been amazing for me, especially hiking, which led to my interest in vortexes. Being in nature is so soothing and grounding. And *crystals*! Y'all, they aren't for everyone, but they are for me. I love flowers, trees, animals, wind, rain, fires, and picking up rocks that need to come home with me. On a nice evening, I find my way to my patio and just read. I love the moon too. It doesn't matter what it is, but doing anything outside helps you to connect with animals, yourself, and others and brings such an internal peace.

Health

Mind, body, and spirit. Sure, no surprise that food and exercise are important, but your health is a culmination of physical, spiritual, mental, and emotional elements. So working to ensure that your body is working well is important. The easiest way to care for yourself is to maintain these—food, sleep, get moving and talking it out. Adding in a great therapist is priceless. Once I found the right one for me, we crushed it in just over one year. We worked through inner child healing, parental issues, shadow work, what irritates me about others and why, relationship styles, and programming and beliefs that no longer agree with me and who I am or who I want to be. Now add in some extra fruits, veggies, daily walks, and meditation and I'm no longer overthinking or refusing to communicate what I need but rather hearing my body loud and clear—most of the time.

Purpose

I've been a chemist for twenty-five years. So when I tell you that I was a logical, square, type A thinker, I am not exaggerating. My purpose is to be a healer. This ability has brought so much life, passion, and excitement out of me that I can barely contain myself some days. When I give a session, I am over the moon.

Let's go back to five years ago, a friend was sitting on my couch, knowing that I'd just changed my whole life, and he asked, "What are you passionate about?" I had no idea. For my whole life, I just thought I was different than other people, that work wasn't meant to make me feel passionate. I mean, I liked it OK, I was good at it, and it paid well, but I just did not have the passionate response these folks had. Well, my friend looked at me horrified. I had no clue at the time that he was launching my quest to be able to answer this question.

Are you ready to begin your quest? Is there one path that calls to you? Do you want something different? Do you want to know what your body feels like when it's working from a healed state?

I suggest beginning with numerology and figuring out what your life path number is. Journaling can be helpful since the healing path is not linear and you may get puzzle pieces today that don't make any sense until months from now. Then work on meditation, and once you get the hang of it, ask your mission animal to visit you. Think about what this animal represents to you. There are plenty of resources to determine the meaning of your mission animal. Look for local classes and resources, or a community to get involved in; there are many ways to approach increasing your intuition and beginning your healing journey.

How do you begin this journey of unweaving the ball of yarn that has collected and twisted since before you were born? You can start by asking your body, mind, and spirit to work with you. Begin to focus on healing and a path for how to begin will start to appear and show you where, how, or who can help you. Setting the intention for healing is critical. Making your healing a priority or a focus is important. Asking questions and searching for direction are key parts to getting started. Many of us know what we want the result to be, but the movement of the path from where we are today to where we want to be is not always clear. This is where your intuition, trust in yourself, and ability to build a good support team as well as a spiritual team come into play. Sometimes we must choose a direction that just feels right even though we cannot yet see the light at the end of the tunnel. Sometimes we will feel lost, confused, and turned around; yet when our higher self is the compass, we are guided, protected, led, and moved in the right direction.

Are you willing to take one step forward, not using logic to guide you but using your highest self who only wants the best for you? I lived my life by using logic only, and I ended up at a dead end. Once I made the choice to start trusting myself, to lean into my intuition, and to focus on letting my higher self guide me, I've found my passion, I've completely changed directions and what I want my life to look like. I've found magic in the day to day and seen amazing things happen. I've dreamed bigger than I ever thought to, and I've not only found how to live in the present but also to build for the future. I no longer live in the logical manner the world taught me to. I want more and bigger things, but they aren't materialistic, and they aren't the typical things. For much of my life I did not even know what I wanted; now my vision is so crystal clear that I am focusing 100 percent of my energy on the knowledge that I am no doubt in the right place, going in the right direction, and with the right guidance. No more asking anyone else if my plan sounds good or right, because how could they know more than I do about what I want and what I need?

What would you do if you could do anything? Some of us no longer know how to dream big. Even if we won a million dollars and could live anywhere, do anything, we'd be lost as to where or what that is. Finding what you are here to do means you don't need a million dollars; you can do something every day that you love. Yes, you may work a job you don't love, but you'll be filled with so much joy that the things and people who drive you crazy will all get quiet. They will still exist, and they likely may not change, but something that festered before will no longer even get a rise out of you.

At one point, I seriously considered leaving the company I'd worked at for over ten years and taking a job that was twice the drive, more work, more travel, and required me to share an office because my workplace had become so frustrating. By using meditation, I realized that while I wanted to leave, my higher self wanted me to stay. If I took the new job, my focus would be proving myself in a new job—working and focusing hard on learning the new job, the people, and the customers. My current job gave me freedom, saved me on driving time, and supplied me with enough funds to allow me to take classes and focus on getting to know me, take part in the community, and open my own business. The value of this was priceless. But how could I stay? The workplace environment was so stressful. Well, some people have come and gone, but the real difference is me. I'm no longer allowing what others are doing, or not doing, to cause my body stress. I focus on controlling the part I am responsible for. I let my supervisor know when I have an issue, and if nothing changes, then it must not be a critical component to the end result.

At the end of day, if I've done my best, the rest is up to the system and the leaders who have been put into place. I get to incorporate what is important to me at work, at home, with my friends, and with my family, and I get to be a happy, healthy part of a community that provides love, support, and checks in on me. A close circle of friends. Well, I never had many friends—you know, without the willingness to be vulnerable and all. But now, I get to call some of the most amazing, loving, supportive, healed people in the world friends. We encourage healing and vulnerability, we accept multiple beliefs, and we are not in competition but cheering for each other. No one is trying to get a bigger bonus, a better rating, or heal the most. Just allowing us to be ourselves in the process of healing, learning as we go, and working together to be amazing.

Chapter 4

LIVING YOUR PURPOSE

Perhaps you are asking if you must quit your job, go back to school, or sell everything you have to live your purpose. Not at all. There are minor changes that you can make that will allow you to begin incorporating each of the healing paths that will help you to find your purpose. Perhaps one way to make small changes is to apply one of the paths a week.

For intuition, perhaps you can ask yourself over your morning coffee, What does my body need today? Then actually listen to what your body needs. This builds intuition and trust with your mind, body, and spirit.

For health, maybe you can consider what foods make you feel good and what foods do not, then continue using how you feel to determine how you eat.

For the conscious/collective, I suggest having compassion. Brene Brown suggests that instead of being frustrated with others, we consider what if this is their best instead of assuming that they are lazy, unintelligent, or not even trying.

For love, how many of our reactions occur out of frustration or because we are trying to protect ourselves. What if instead of shutting down when we feel vulnerable, we open up further?

Nature, I think, is sometimes the easiest. Just sit outside for a few moments or even take off your shoes and step onto the grass. What about buying yourself flowers or watching birds at a feeder? All these things involve stopping for just a few moments and connecting with someone or our surroundings. These things allow you to stop and take a moment prior to giving your reaction. This allows you to be present and take a few breaths.

The world we live in is moving at such a pace that there are so many things we can miss if we are focused on getting there or checking a box instead of the process or space between start and finish. The destination is important, but life happens from here to there—look at how much you miss if the arrival point is the only one you take in. Imagine only hearing the last twenty seconds of a song or the last twenty minutes of a movie, all the pieces that build up to the finale. If that's all you experience, when do you learn to pull for the characters, see and understand their struggles, or consider what you would like to happen? Just like all your experiences combine to make you who you are, your experiences all help you with your purpose. You gain the experience that helps you with your purpose, helps you decide what you like and don't, where you want to live, and the kinds of people you want to spend your time with. Living helps you make decisions. Finding your purpose is a decision. Living your purpose is a decision. Healing is a decision.

I decided that something had to change. Decisions had to be made another way. Logic had not gotten me to where I had hoped to go. I had rolled the wrong combination of dice and took the slide back twenty spaces. So as I had an opportunity to experience those twenty spaces (or years, in my case) another way, did I want to continue the method and approach that had gotten me to this place, or was there something else to try?

I knew that something about me had put me in this place and while I was unsure of the way to do it differently, I did realize that exploring it was critical. While I spent time in therapy, I continued to ask what led me to spend almost twenty years in a situation that was so unhealthy. Knowing that the answer was within myself, I continued to ask that we focus on me and what was going on with me. And finally the right therapist asked me what my attachment style was. This term, being completely new to me, was the crack in the shell.

Now, I'm not saying the other therapists had not been helpful, but we were not getting to the roots of the issue. See, I've already lived over forty years of life experiences, and some of my calculations of events were distorted;

some of my thought processes were built from trauma and unhealthy experiences. Through therapy with the right therapist, I learned to explore my inner child, shadow work, parental relationships, past relationships, and experiences that built the framework for my current belief system. This indicated that my decision-making skills needed review.

Many of the things that I believed about myself, men, and love had been the result of unhealthy situations. Based on my own analysis, I had drawn conclusions or made rules based on poor data. Our bodies are amazing systems, but sometimes the programs we are running need to be updated or defragmented. When our body does not work properly, instead of being frustrated at our bodies, we should ask ourselves, Why is my body doing this? What is it trying to tell me? What does my body need?

On this path, I've learned so much about my body, whom I'd not been working well with for several years; it had been throwing red flags, and I'd been ignoring them.

Six years ago, I was diagnosed with SIBO (small intestinal bacterial overgrowth) after a year of painful symptoms associated with foods. I was told that SIBO is untreatable and, therefore, I had to eliminate the triggering foods from my diet completely. As I learned new healing tools, I'd tried them all to remove SIBO from my body, without success. Then a friend, the owner of Indiglow Soul, mentioned the importance of understanding why and when my body developed this sickness and understanding what it does for me or what it protects me from.

What a game changer.

I simply had a conversation with my body to understand what it was trying to say to me. My body was trying to ask me how many of the things that I loved I would have to lose to do something about it. And little by little, my life and my marriage at the time were shutting down. Now I'd even lost my favorite foods. I listened to my body, thanked it for the message, released it, and began eating all the foods I'd been avoiding for six years with no symptoms.

Why do we treat sickness like a failure instead of asking what the message is? My body was trying to communicate, protect, and even help. Understanding the symbolism or the message can be more complicated, but it's not when you love yourself, trust yourself, and listen to your body. Our body is an amazing tool that has the ability to heal, if we tap into it. I've now gone through all my concerns with my body to understand and release them. What is your body trying to tell you?

What stops us from working toward healing or wanting to heal? Comfort? Not knowing where to start? Our self-esteem? Family or friend dynamics? Yes, all of that certainly makes it more difficult. Many times in my life, I've had the thought that if I could just hide on an abandoned island (a well taken care of resort is preferred) for a month and completely disconnect from all people, TV, and responsibilities that I would be able to figure out some things. Well, I was never able to do that, but moving to a one-bedroom apartment with little furniture, no chores to do, and living alone certainly helped. That doesn't stop work, bills, and constant thinking. So what is it? I think it is one small reoccurring thought that something needs to change, then putting your body in that direction and moving one step at a time. My body was so overloaded by the time I took my step that I felt like a fish out of water. I don't recommend or encourage you to pick up and leave everything. I suggest that people listen to their bodies. I had ignored mine for so many years that I did not even know what my body was saying. Is your body sick or healing? Do you feel frustrated or content? Are you happy or just going through the motions? Are you living?

What does living mean? Sure, you are breathing and moving. Maybe you have a family, a home, which is surely living, right? Is it? Life sometimes feels like a hamster wheel. You get up, take a shower, go to work, exercise, dinner, sleep, and repeat. Is that a life worth living? Well, sure. But what if at the end of each day you could take three minutes to recap with gratitude the most important moments of the day?

Since being on this journey, I love saying out loud the recap of my day. I usually say something like "You know, typical day—saved a dog, cleansed and cleared a house, sent a spirit to the light, and had a PB and J sandwich."

It reminds me that life is simple, amazing, and magical. Yeah, I also did the hamster wheel stuff too, but there were beautiful moments that made this day special.

Are you on the hamster wheel? What is one thing you could do to set today apart from every other day? Watch a movie with a child, have coffee with a neighbor, or call a friend who you've been too busy to talk to. These are the moments that bring joy, fulfillment, wonder, creativity, enjoyment, and connection. All these work toward understanding others, building relationships, and becoming present. We've all heard the saying "your presence *is* the present," and that is so true! I know that many days, I was just going through the motions and I could not have even described what my husband was wearing had he been kidnapped. Seriously, my eyes were not even working. I was on autopilot. Is life about being on autopilot? Hell no! Ever hear the phrase "stop and smell the roses"? That's what we are supposed to be doing. If we are moving so fast that we miss seeing the journey, we really miss so many of the good parts. When we take time to slow down, process, absorb, focus, listen, and enjoy, what a delight it is.

So where in a busy life does healing take place? First, know that when healing is happening, you are becoming a better parent, friend, sibling, person, and so on anytime you are incorporating time for healing, so every minute you dedicate to healing is totally worth it.

I like first thing in the morning, when the world is quiet

and I'm having a cup of coffee. Everything is slow and calm. But you can dedicate time to healing while you are brushing your teeth, in the shower, at lunch, or during a yoga class. It can also be during meditation, therapy, or with someone trained in healing. But it truly is something as simple as sitting outside for a few minutes, being present, and listening to nature and your body.

Do you ever think about what you would do differently if you could start over? Each day is an opportunity to begin again, react differently, make a new decision, and look at the same problem through a new viewpoint. Proactive healing does just that—allows you to recalculate, think differently, choose another path, stop doing it the same way you always have.

What if you reviewed how yesterday went and just picked out one or two things that you could do a new way? Would you have picked another meal at the restaurant? Would you respond nicer to a person at the store who cut you off at the grocery line? I am not recommending regretting or pining over all the things that you did wrong or right but rather simply choosing to improve upon your experience.

My back used to be so tight, my jaw clenched, and I'd even leave nail marks on my palms when I slept because my hands would be in a ball. Looking back, all the tension, stress, frustration, and disappointment were a result of refusing to have the hard conversations and struggling to make decisions that I knew had to be made, all because of the confusion I felt from my own wounds and no understanding of my partner's wounds. Imagine if the two of us had talked, worked through our own trauma and relationship issues, and at least were able to have a discussion that was from a healed place. After working on myself, I realized that most of the fights we had were about trying to win or be right when, if we had just held hands and walked together in the same direction, the result of any fight would have been completely different.

Why did I need to be right? Why couldn't I see the pain that he brought to the relationship? Because I was so busy trying to not see my own, trying to keep it all together, trying to not rock the boat, trying to people please, and trying to navigate life while ignoring any of the things I had never dealt with. And to be even more honest, I didn't even know I had trauma or issues. I did not even realize that I was operating from an unhealed place. If I had been asked, I'd have said, "I have no reason to visit a therapist."

Here's where I remind you that I have been on a healing journey for over five years, and I've been in therapy the entire time. So guess what? If everyone around you needs healing, chances are you do too. And it turns out that some of my issues were not things that people did or said to me but rather their thoughts and how I reacted being an empath. Based on what I took in for so many years without the protection of my energy,

I'd stored so many memories and emotions that my body would excessively sweat to try to eliminate the toxins. I'd been so mad at my body since I was a child because sweating kept me from being close to people, touching people, being comfortable in social situations, but it turns out that it was my body's protection mechanism because I'm an empath. Imagine if my body had not been sweating to help with the removal of toxins. Being on a healing journey has taught me to heal my body instead of beating my body up for not being normal.

Your body is a magical being. It houses all your systems and organs, and it is built to self-heal. This system works much better when it is properly taken care of. What do I mean by that? Well, what you feed it is extremely important. By feeding it, I don't just mean your stomach. Your body needs a physically, mentally, emotionally, and spiritually safe environment to thrive and heal.

So we begin with what we feed out bodies: food. Sounds simple enough, but is it? We often eat foods that are not good for us, have little nutrition, are low-vibration foods, or our body does not like. If your body bloats, hurts, or reacts negatively to the food you eat that is your body telling you this food should be avoided or there is something to further investigate. So many people simply eat what they like and ignore the side effects. Eating intuitively and taking the time to figure out how your body feels when you eat something, is a great way to listen to your body.

What do you feed your mind? The people in your circle, your home environment, the music you listen to, the books you read, the shows and movies you watch, and even the conversations you have with yourself and others are the foods you are feeding your mind. Your thoughts are energy. They are stored in your body and can cause health issues. What fuel is your mind absorbing?

How in the world do you feed your spirit? By doing things that bring you joy, excitement, laughter, peace, calmness, and love. Your body needs to be safe on the outside and on the inside as it houses the most amazing person—*you*. You are your mind, body, and spirit, and all these parts play a role in your health and wellbeing. Your body, when fed properly, works so much better to heal. If you begin to listen to your body, you will realize that any the parts that aren't working right are signals. These signals are trying to get your attention, because there is something in your mind, body, or spirit that is asking for attention. When you are experiencing pain that is not only physical, ask yourself, What is this trying to tell me? What do I need to know? The answers to these questions can be profound, you may even be amazed by your own body, and even after you've been in this same body for so many years, you will think you've met the most intelligent stranger, but it's still your body. Instead of being frustrated, be curious. What does this disease teach me? Why did my body need this disease? What does my body need to communicate?

What about self-love? How many folks think of a bath or a mani-pedi? These are not the solutions at all. Self-love is about how you talk to yourself, treat yourself, listen to yourself, and trust yourself. I don't know about you, but I've likely let myself down more than others have. I've had conversations with myself multiple times, trying to give myself the rules, making promises and deals, only to find out I wasn't a very trustworthy friend to myself, so I had to do some big work to get back trust. I still work on it daily. If a simple task kicks my ass, I immediately tear myself down. That's not very constructive since I'd never say those things to other people.

The way someone once described it to me was to imagine growing a big, beautiful tree and admiring this tree, then stepping back, picking up an ax, and whacking at the truck of the tree. Well, that is what we do to ourselves when we don't have self-love. We aren't stupid or dumb; we are human, and we make mistakes, which we learn and grow from.

I can recall the day that I realized I finally loved myself. I had an epiphany. Instead of expecting anything from another, I simply said out loud, "I need to be a refuge for myself. I need to hear and listen to myself. I need to keep my word to myself. I need to take care of myself. I need to provide a safe, secure, and loving place for myself."

Wow! No matter how many times I've revisited this statement, it still makes me cry when I say it out loud.

Now when I hear myself chopping at my trunk, I call

myself out. Out loud, I say, "Stop it! This is not helpful." I'm not perfect, but I'm trying. Self-love supplies a safe place for you (mind, body, and spirit). When things are going wrong, I need to support myself, not add to the pile.

Can you imagine feeding your body all these ways, plus fully embracing all of yourself, even the parts of your body and personality you don't love? Can you imagine how peaceful your body systems would feel? I'm practically relaxing just thinking about it. As I write this morning after my walk, I'm just sitting outside in the breeze. Nowhere to be, just being. If just being the you that you truly are is possible, what would be the purpose of being anyone else?

As kids, we are often asked, What do you want to be when you grow up? Tell me your dreams. If you could be or do anything, what would it be? Some kids may even have heard that they could be anything they want to be. And somewhere between those comments and questions is where we often get derailed. Then only when you lose a job/get divorced do people start to ask those questions again.

It happened to me in 2009. I had worked one job for eleven years, since college. My job sent us to a career center. They offered tests to find your skills and preferences as well as classes to help hone your skills. During this time of so much pressure to pay my bills, people just kept saying, This is your opportunity to do anything! What do you want to do? Uh, I want to make money, I want to give you the finger, and I want to cry.

This opportunity did not feel exciting, thrilling, or like having a dream come true. It felt like a nightmare. I was on a tight budget. I had to redefine who I was and figure out if my skills were transferable to any other job. Were they? Well, yes, it took a while, and the new job was way different, and my paycheck was cut in half, but let me tell you what I learned during those eighteen months. I learned to hustle, to talk to strangers, to network, and to sell myself.

Fast forward and these skills are still working for me today, and I've applied them to my personal business. OK, so while I had zero clue what dream I wanted to fulfill in 2009, I totally figured it out in 2023. Sometimes we have no idea why we are going through the experiences that we are at the time, but we can easily see how many of those are strung together to give us the background we need to survive future experiences. Life is like that. We have a path in mind, and sometimes it looks like we got diverted or lost, but did we? Life and healing have a lot in common but rarely are the route with the shortest distance to the end destination.

Why do we worry so much about the destination or end point? We laser focus on the results of everything as if the results bring all the joy. Have you ever made a list of the things that bring you joy? I'd be shocked if many or any of them look like results or destinations.

Make a list of ten things that bring you joy.

1.

2.

3.

4.

5.

6.

7.

8.

9.

10.

What is joy? When I made my list and meditated on joy, I found most of them were simple and small. It is tiny moments that I find pleasure in. These moments cause me to pause as if surprised, almost amused, and then a smile will cross my face. These aren't the kind of surprises that cause your body to become energized but rather to sink or ground into the present moment. When I notice joy in my body I am humming.

I love to cook. I love the smells and the anticipation. I love having another person taste my dish and being the one to see the changes in their expression. I love the noises people make when they truly enjoy something they are eating. I know I'm joyful when I hear myself hum. I'm happy, content, relaxed, and enjoying what I am doing at this moment. We don't do enough of the things that bring us joy, and we need to begin finding ways to bring joy into everyday life stuff.

Can joy be chased? I don't think so. I do think you can be intentional about it by choosing not to rush through the everyday. There is so much magic in every day. But certainly, knowing what you find joy in and incorporating those elements is important. I like to cook, but there are many ways that I can cook. I can rush through it, frustrated and attempting to cross one more thing off my list, followed by mindless eating while watching TV. Or I can light a candle and slow down, taking in the smells, being creative with the dish I'm making, and being in the moment while I eat. The difference in these two approaches is about fifteen minutes, but they are completely different experiences for my entire system. We think sometimes that if we can complete the to-do list and just finish (fill in the blank), then we can relax and enjoy life. With that thought process, life is passing you by.

Let's go deeper onto the healing paths. Let's begin with nature. You can live in a high-rise and still experience nature. Consider a walk in a local park, buy an indoor plant, or listen to nature music, like ocean or rainforest sounds. Nature connects you to the earth, animals, plants, rocks, and everything else around us. It brings a grounding presence and roots us firmly in the present. When it snows and everything is covered in white, have you ever noticed how time slows down, life feels quiet, calm, peaceful, and it almost snuggles you? Think about all the different seasons and possible weather conditions and how they bring different energy.

What about baby season? Baby animals. Bird nests everywhere, a mother goose with her babies following— spring coming in. Each season brings with it different colors, temperatures, rituals, and things that you can look forward to. Walking on the beach. Hearing the ocean as it moves in and out. Feeling the sand on your bare feet. Nature is powerful. It contains the elements of earth, wind, fire, and water. You have the four seasons: spring, summer, fall, and winter. You have the mountains and the oceans and the deserts. This grounding leads to acknowledgment of nature, which tends to pull you in and connect you. Then there is an appreciation and gratitude.

How can you bring nature into your everyday life? What seasons and elements are you drawn to? If nature is the healing path that you resonate the most with, you may even find that your work includes nature. There are many ways to incorporate loving nature into everyday life, like as a marine biologist or science teacher, working or volunteering with park services, or just being a lover of crystals. You may even find that nature (earth and grounding) is a great fit to help round out your astrological chart.

I also love doing yard work—pulling weeds, gardening, and even picking up sticks. I used to rush through my chores to get to something else and always found myself too tired to do anything. When I moved from a house to an apartment, I was desperate to do something outside. Don't laugh, but I even pulled weeds at the apartment when no one was looking. I ended up learning that I love hiking and indoor plants. I also found time to sit on my third-floor balcony, listening to nature and watching sunsets and the moon. I needed nature to heal.

Water has become such a crucial element for me. My chart has a lot of fire, air, and earth with very little water. I have always loved sitting by the ocean and hearing it; I once even slept with the door open in a hotel room just to hear the ocean all night. My damaged system craved water for relaxation and healing. Lots of baths and showers, enjoying the rain, sitting by water, and even making friends with people who had a lot of water in their charts. Feeling people who felt calm like water was one of the first energies I could feel. Water represents emotions. My emotions, other than frustration and anger, had been turned off for a long time. When I started to heal, I began to cry (water). Water has ended up being such an important piece to my healing that I created Healing Waters.

Today, I do yard work in smaller pieces and at a much slower pace. One of my favorite things to do is walk around the yard to pick up sticks or pull a few weeds. Often when I am reading or writing, I'm sitting outside. I've even made a little oasis in my garage for when it is raining or too hot. I have a collection of crystals inside and many rocks that I've collected from hikes outside. Nature helped me heal and find joy.

SHELLY R. FOX

Think of ten ways you can enjoy nature or incorporate nature into your everyday life.

1.

2.

3.

4.

5.

6.

7.

8.

9.

10.

What do we have if we do not have our health? Health is so important, and we must begin to heal by using the amazing body that we have been given. We often believe that our body is failing us somehow by the aches, pains, and symptoms we experience. But what if our body has been trying to communicate and we have not been able to receive the messages? Our body has many complicated organ systems and an entire nervous system, which appears to work and repair itself for the most part. We have one body, so it makes sense to care about our health.

The health of your body should really be thought about in terms of mind, body, and spirit. Complete health needs to consider physical, emotional, mental, and spiritual elements. The most common tools associated with health are diet and exercise, and yes, those are very important, but there is so much more. By the time we become adults, most of us have experienced many interactions with other people. These can be positive or negative and can force us to experience happy, sad, and a hundred other emotions. Depending upon the environment we grew up in and the parents we were born to, we have several experiences that either we did not know how to process or may have only processed to the best of our ability at the time.

I want to break down the different elements of health mentioned in this section.

Physical

The basics here are diet, exercise, and general caring for your physical body. My big rule of thumb is to not ignore physical symptoms and to do some of the already mentioned basics. Sleep is a critical piece of your body's capability to heal. I'm no specialist, but here's my suggestion: plan for the sleep your body needs. Eat what makes you feel good, and don't eat what your body appears to disagree with. Move every day in some way (exercise). Rest when your body says it needs to rest. Play lots. Play can connect you to your childhood and can also be a great gateway to joy.

I do not compromise my sleep. My entire life revolves around my need for sleep at night. This is one of what my therapist would refer to as non-negotiables. I eat intuitively, meaning that I change and plan my diet based on what I hear through meditation and intuition. I've been primarily a vegetarian for about two years now and have removed other foods for periods of time, but eating intuitively also allows me to eat without stressing over it.

I generally like to combine nature and exercise, but the weather does not always allow that. But I'm a walker, a slow walker, but I walk most days. I often feel guilty about resting, but do not feel guilty about taking care of your body. I've gotten better; when I hear to rest, I generally can do so without too much guilt.

Play is the most challenging one for me personally. I

love to have fun, but I find this one comes less naturally for me. I often feel like I must think about what I can incorporate into my day that feels fun, especially if I'm on a budget. Some ways that I've brought in play include going to an ice cream shop, painting, crafts, and watching children's movies.

Emotional

Emotions are healthy. Most of us can't even name what emotions we are feeling. For this, I highly recommend *Atlas of the Heart* by Brene Brown. Yes, I love Brene Brown, if you haven't figured that out yet. Our use of emotional language is so limited. We often improperly label the emotion we are experiencing. On top of that, there are many emotions that we do not know how to process or because of timing and place, can't properly process. This is where healing modalities like Emotion Code, Body Code and removal of heart walls come into play. Some of the most important parts of my personal healing journey required me to pause for a few minutes, and sometimes a few days, to really think about what I was feeling. So many times, I leaned on anger, frustration, and irritation when I really felt hurt, embarrassment, and absolute brokenness, but my ego did not want to let another person know that they had made me feel that way. ow your emotions play into your health really revolves around understanding what emotions you are

SHELLY R. FOX

truly feeling and then experiencing them. The second part is learning what role they play in your health and how to address them.

Mental

So the most obvious answer here is a therapist, and I do believe this is a vital part of a healing journey. I doubt that many of us have become adults and managed to avoid trauma or experiences that have created our reality with a slightly skewed viewpoint. There is inner-child work, work with parents and family members, any relationships, and then all your experiences, positive and negative. Two other important pieces are shadow work and all the people and things that drive you mad. Who are you jealous of? What do you judge yourself for? What parts of yourself do you like and dislike? For me, I found that I have a lot of traits that are, in fact, opposites. I am a rule follower, but I also really like bucking the system—this is an example of a shadow.

There is a lot to unpack here, but I can tell you that it is totally worth it. This will improve all your relationships— the most important one with yourself, but also with your family, friends, and coworkers. Understanding yourself is more than half the battle. Once you understand who you are, what you need, and what has come together to create you, it changes everything. There is not another person anywhere who has the same story and experiences. This makes you unique, special, and complicated. Thoughts are energy, as we've previously discussed, so how you think/talk to yourself is a big factor in your mental health. All the conversations you have with yourself—sure, no one else hears them, but the most important person does: *you*.

Spiritual

Who are you, and what do you believe? I don't mean what you grew up believing or what you are supposed to believe. I mean, question everything. My entire life, I accepted what I was taught. At some point in the last ten years, I did start to ask a few questions about religion but also just kept trying harder to believe, accept, and get as excited as I saw other people on their religious journeys. I even thought that I just wasn't as excited or wasn't a passionate person or that I was doing something wrong. Finally, when I started questioning everything after my divorce, I got around to asking myself, What do I believe is right and wrong? What does a higher power mean for me?

For me, one of the most beautiful things in my journey is understanding that my belief system does not include someone else deciding what is right and wrong for me; my mind, body, and spirit decide what is acceptable for me. I am no longer religious, but I am the most spiritual and passionate that I've ever been in my entire life. I mediate every day. I feel connected to my body, plants, animals, and others and have a sense of community and compassion for others that I've never experienced. When something does not go as I'd hoped, I try to understand how I can use what I know to help next time. This leads me to one of my favorite learnings.

For those working on a spiritual journey, the term "higher self" is common. It refers to your highest good without ego. I focused on following this for the last year and realized that my body was not working at its highest potential. For this reason, my mind (mental), body (emotions, physical body), and spirit (highest self) need to be in agreement for the peace of my entire being. My physical body and mind don't always accept the highest and best perspective of myself. So after a few confused moments, this is the approach that I will be trying next for myself and clients.

Think of ten ways that these four elements could be a part of your healing journey

1.

2.

3.

4.

5.

6.

7.

8.

9.

10.

Let me give you some examples. A woman has physical symptoms of an autoimmune disorder. She goes to the doctor, and they set up tests and prescriptions. She also wants to consider her other options. The energy healer she visits believes the woman does not have an autoimmune disease but certainly has the symptoms of one and that her body wants her attention. The energy healer believes it is emotional and spiritual, then suggests including meditation while working to understand the lesson her body is trying to teach her. The woman's body does not feel good, and it is in pain and wants relief as quickly as possible. Her mind wants to take the medicine from the doctor because she is afraid that things will get worse. Her spirit wants to believe in energy healing and work on it. What should she do? To bring her body, mind, and spirit together for a plan, she cautiously takes the medicine, aware of possible side effects to her digestive system. Her body takes rest. She reduces the activities she has planned for the next few weeks, then she plans to meditate and work on what she hears.

The same goes with other treatments, like cancer treatment; healing should include many approaches. I think using all your resources is a more well-rounded approach and leads to a full recovery as well as peace of the mind, body, and spirit. It simply takes your entire system into account.

I recommend getting to know the six healing paths.

All the healing paths are important to include on your healing journey. They each have aspects that reconnect us to ourselves and to each other. Becoming present and connected are key elements to rediscovering who you are and who you want to be.

Intuition

Some of us have a feeling, some a knowing, some see or have dreams, while some hear messages. All of these ways and others are simply a result of being connected to your body and listening. When you are connected to your body and aware of what your body needs, it's easy, but so many of us are not connected to our bodies.

Our body sends signals and messages, but being present and being willing to listen is critical. Many of us experience déjà vu, or encounter a dream that we believe has meaning. Being willing to explore the meaning and trust the direction provided is not always easy because it often goes against our logic and teachings.

Once you tune into your body and begin to listen, you can hear messages that direct you to rest, sleep, play, and food/drink. All these things can give the body what it needs and provide healing.

For the people whom intuition is the primary healing type, this can involve Reiki, hands-on healing, or energy, or careers in emergency response and hospice. For others, it can be a meditation practice or learning to work with their intuition and higher self, working to connect the spirit with mind and body.

Love

Many of us say I love you, but the true meaning has been lost. The same goes for self-love. It seems to be diluted down to bubble baths and self-care routines. Love is about first accepting yourself, becoming a safe place, a refuge for yourself and making sure that you learn to set boundaries and ask for what you need to ensure that you can trust and rely on yourself. A great way to determine what you are not providing for yourself is to determine what you feel others never get right. For example, it may be that they never listen to you and what you need— most likely, the reality is that *you* do not listen to yourself and what you need. Once you begin to listen to yourself, others will follow your lead.

Love is also unconditional. Meaning you love yourself even if you need to lose a few pounds or you make mistakes. Many of us have heard the phrase "if you wouldn't say it to a friend, why would you say it to yourself." Self-love and loving others can be so healing. It means that a healthy relationship with yourself first leads to much healing. Unconditionally loving others without expectation is a hard ask, but it can be rewarding.

The typical jobs or roles where love is the primary healing type can include a yoga practitioner, a dietitian, a massage therapist, an elementary school teacher, or just a person who has overcome many obstacles in the path to appreciating their body. Choosing to focus on giving and receiving love leads to joy. Love opens great possibilities and welcomes so many of the emotions that can sometimes feel elusive, like joy, elation, and euphoria.

For some, love can be the most difficult because it does require vulnerability and courage and many of us have built up walls and armor to protect ourselves when "love" hasn't gone our way, but if we can understand what has caused the fear, the trust issues, and has prevented us from being vulnerable, we can love ourselves so much more and in turn, love others more as well.

Conscious/Collective

How many of us are concerned about the world around us, and how many of us are oblivious to the world around us? If you are one of the people, whose heart strings get tugged while watching many of the events happening around the world and feel like there is something you can do, this is likely where you find the most healing.

Community events, potlucks, festivals, group activities, men's/women's circles, schools, churches, or organizations. If you meditate, then even your messages likely apply to more than just yourself, and it is important for you to share them with others.

This type of healing calls you to be with others, help

others, and improve your community. Not only does it help you but it greatly helps those around you, and it spreads. This can sometimes feel like a big task since you are balancing yourself and giving so much to others.

Nature

Witnessing spring, the first snow, a good cleansing rain, a walk in the woods, or simply visiting a zoo. Nature reminds us that we must learn to let go like the leaves and that every season has its purpose. Your life also tends to have seasons. We learn to plant seeds and wait for them to grow. If we spend time in nature, we can also connect more to ourselves, animals, plants, and the earth.

Connection is vital to fully appreciating life and all it has to offer. Nature brings connection, relaxation, grounding, and healing.

Perhaps walking or hiking soothes you, or listening to the ocean come in and out. Maybe bird-watching, or even working as a guide at a park soothes you. Consider what brings you peace and how you use nature, the elements, the weather, or the seasons to lead you.

Health

The connection of mind, body, and spirit is such a vital one. Your health is not one function but many: physical, mental, emotional, and spiritual, and how they interact and play together. It is extremely important to understand and ensure that basic health needs like food, water, sleep, and shelter are met, but there is so much more to health.

How do you talk to yourself? How do you set boundaries with others? Are you mindful and present? Do you listen to your body when it tells you what it needs? Are you willing to give that to your body?

Movement is also a big part of health. It could be exercise, yoga, dancing, or walking in nature. It could also be the company you keep. How do those around you affect your health and well-being? When you focus on what your body, mind, and spirit need, you are in a good place for yourself and able to determine better what you can and can't do for others.

Ways to incorporate health include self-love understanding, studying yoga, researching the mind/body connection, going to a therapist, or being a therapist. Health, like all the other healing paths, has many aspects and each person can certainly find something that feels authentic and comfortable to incorporate.

Purpose

What is your purpose? What are you passionate about?

Some of us figure it out when we are children, and we know exactly what we want to do for a career, for hobbies, or what we want our life to look like. Others take a little longer; for me, I was over forty and looking for my purpose and what I was passionate about. It took my life—the one I'd built to exact specifications, falling apart for me to reevaluate my life, values, and focus and to determine what was important. I felt like such a failure when I would be asked, "What are you passionate about?" At forty-two, in the middle of a divorce, sitting in my apartment with barely any furniture, I had no idea. It certainly wasn't the life I'd built or the job I had. I wasn't a wife, a mother, a homeowner, or anything I had aspired to for the last twenty-plus years. I'd never felt passionate about much.

What does purpose give you? Direction. Happiness. Focus. And it can act as a compass for your entire life. If you have loved art since you were a kid, and have always put it off and miss it, guess what your purpose is? For my friend who asked me about my passion, his is art—and within his art, to communicate with others. Your purpose can be anything; it can lead to a career, a hobby, a family, and it can drive how you spend your time. You may have to experiment to figure it out, but follow what interests you, where you are curious, where it doesn't feel like a chore, and where you feel energized, not exhausted. There you most certainly are going in the right direction.

Chapter 5

SPREADING THE LIGHT

No matter which of the healing paths you use, any healing that you do for yourself spreads. It moves throughout your life and the lives of your family and friends, your coworkers, and even those who have passed and those who have yet to arrive.

Even a candle in the darkest of rooms adds a lot of light. Hence *Finding your Light*. I certainly believe that I was living in the dark, missing out on some of the most beautiful of moments, but also just so barricaded behind protection that I was not really living. I was alive, and from the outside, I seemed to be hitting all the marks in life, but I was not passionate, I did not know who I was, and I felt lost and alone, numb. To remove the conditioning and protection that I'd spent my entire life building up in order to ensure that I did not make mistakes, have failures, or get hurt did not prevent any of that from happening. As the onion analogy goes, the layers were getting peeled back. I did not even know who I was, what I needed, what

I wanted, or what had gotten me to this place. As I started to explore healing via intuition, each step would send me searching, questioning, and trying to answer some of those questions.

Again, healing is not linear, and it is not logical. But as I reflect on the last five years of my healing journey, I know myself better than ever. I know my purpose is to help others find their light and to continue to work through removing all the protection I no longer need. I enjoy sitting on my patio, drinking a cup of coffee, and often I even walk slower, enjoying the journey. I weave myself through the different types of healing depending on the topic of the day.

So what is light? Light is what guides you, moves you, makes you smile, brings you to life, finds who you really are, and finds who you were meant to be. It sets you on fire, it lights you up, it excites you, and it drives you. It's living life in the moment, being present, feeling your body, and connecting with others and the world around you. It's contagious, it spreads, and it changes your perspective.

It's important to understand self-love better. Self-love was a strange concept for me, even after several years of therapy. I was confident as a child/young adult, and even as I'd aged, if I compared myself to others around me, I seemed more comfortable with my body than most. I also felt I did a pretty good job of taking care of myself: diet, exercise, sleep, showers, hair, makeup, ironing my clothes, doing great at my job, and even painting my toenails each week. As it turns out, that had very little to do with how much I took care of myself. I needed to learn to ask for what I needed, to set boundaries, and to do all the things that I'd been mad at others for not doing.

So many times, I had said that I just wanted someone to hear me, see me, love me, listen to me, and be there for me. Why were so many people untrustworthy? Well, I'd not been listening to myself for years. I'd made myself so many promises I did not keep. I'd not been someone I could trust as I'd set ground rules for myself and others and then during the situation, completely let myself down.

As it turns out, I had more than one reason for these things. A parent I couldn't trust, a desire to people please, a thought process that I needed to have value to those who could possibly love me, and I'm an empath. Because I am an empath, I commonly let the needs of others supersede my own. So much so that asking for what I needed felt like the hardest thing in the world because I had associated asking for what I need with losing and disappointing people.

Self-Love for me includes taking care of my physical needs and ensuring that I listen to my body when it talks. But it also includes not tearing myself down when I fail or something doesn't go as planned. Setting better boundaries so I don't feel taken advantage of is also important. I needed to keep my word to myself so I could learn to trust. I needed to hear myself and listen. I needed to be a refuge for *myself*. I needed to be there for *myself*.

I need to love myself so much that I protect myself. I needed to learn to listen to my body and my intuition about others so I could watch out for myself. Self-love is not a bubble bath; sometimes it is, but not being one of the voices that destroys the beautiful person I have been discovering is the biggest piece.

One of the most beautiful people I know put it this way: imagine the most beautiful tree that you have been caring for and then taking an axe to it. Your words do just that. I was the one who could not trust myself, so I could not trust others. I did not believe I was worthy of unconditional love. It was my voice that was the toughest on me and could inflict the most damage.

I work on this every day, and if this is the only part of your healing that you work on, it's totally worth it as this will change your perspective of the world, yourself, and will influence those around you. Loving yourself is the best gift you can give to yourself and the world. There is only one of you—unique, special, and beautiful. Your body does amazing things. Be grateful.

Printed in the USA
CPSIA information can be obtained
at www.ICGtesting.com
LVHW021333110924
790643LV00014B/912

9 798765 252536